The Hair Loss Handbook

BEN CRADDOCK

ISBN: **1494312964**
ISBN-13: **978-1494312961**

DISCLAIMER

The information in this book is based solely on the author's research. While every effort has been taken to ensure the information provided is correct, the content does not constitute medical advice and should not be taken as such. Any medical concerns should be taken up with your doctor prior to the commencement of any treatment discussed in this book.

CONTENTS

1 INTRODUCTION

Before I get into any sort of detail, I'd like to first explain a bit about my experience of hair loss and why I decided to write this book...

When I was around nineteen years old, I noticed my hairline beginning to recede. I had known from an early age that I was likely to lose my hair as I have never known my dad to be anything other than bald, but had always thought of it as being 'one of those things that happens when you get older'. Actually seeing it begin to happen at a time of my life when appearances were one of my main priorities, however, made the harsh reality of it kick in.

By the time I was twenty one, I had become ever-conscious of my continually receding hairline, and had also noticed the hair on the crown of my head becoming much thinner. This consumed a lot more of my thoughts than I would let on, and actually made me quite depressed at certain points in time. Like most people, particularly at the time, I was unaware of any genuine treatments for hair loss and considered baldness to be an inevitability.

While some people appear to be able to accept the balding process, I could not even begin to do this. I felt like I was losing a part of my identity, a part of me. Besides, I knew from times previously when I had had my hair cut short that I didn't have the right shape of head to consider shaving it off. And the idea of having a 'comb-over' in my twenties didn't really appeal to me much either!

Bored at home one day, I decided to investigate the subject online, to see how other people coped with their hair loss. It didn't take long before the brand name 'Rogaine' (or 'Regaine' in the UK) came up. Researching this a bit further, I was excited to discover that this product could not only prevent further hair loss, but actually re-grow some hair that had already fallen out! Suddenly there was a glimmer of hope.

This set me off on a mission that lasted years – and, to an extent, still continues to this day. I spent hours at a time reading everything I could about potential solutions for hair loss, from countless sources. I tried a great number of products in order to see for myself which ones worked and which didn't. As a result I regained a full head of hair and, at the age of thirty, I'm very happy to say that it's all still there!

Over the years of researching the subject, I've been shocked to discover how little useful information there is out there. Almost every website you go to that appears to be giving unbiased information is generally trying to push a particular product in order to gain some affiliate commission from doing so. Often without any regard for the efficacy of the product they are trying to sell you.

I created this ebook in response to this, as I believe there is a need for a factual look at the best ways to combat hair loss, based on unbiased experience. I hope you will find the information here useful, and wish you success on your journey to re-growing and retaining a full head of hair!

2 THE GROWTH CYCLE

Although the term 'hair loss' is usually used to refer to the process of going bald, in actual fact hair loss is actually a completely normal and healthy occurrence.

In fact, we all lose some hair every day of our lives. This is because of the way in which the growth cycle works.

There are 3 phases which make up the growth cycle of hair on the scalp:

Anagen Phase

Most people's scalp contains between 100,000 and 150,000 hair follicles. At any one time, around 95% of these are actively growing. This is known as the Anagen phase. Hair follicles usually remain in this phase for about two and a half years.

Catagen Phase

When a hair follicle reaches then end of the Anagen phase, it enters the Catagen phase. This is where the hair stops growing. This phase only lasts for around two weeks.

Telogen Phase

After the Catagen phase, the hair follicle moves into the Telogen phase, also known as the resting phase. During this phase, the follicle becomes completely inactive and the hair will fall out. Hair follicles remain in this phase for around three months before moving back into the Anagen phase.

Many people are unaware of the growth cycle and therefore panic when they wake up with hair on their pillow, or discover excessive amounts of hair stuck to their hair brush.

As there is no way of predicting exactly when each follicle is going to enter any particular phase, there will be times when more follicles will be in the Telogen phase than usual, and therefore more hair is lost than normal. This can give the illusion of there being a hair loss problem, when in actual fact any lost hair will soon grow back.

For this reason I felt it important to make you aware of how the growth cycle works in order for you to first eliminate this as a possible cause before moving on to treatment.

3 WHY DO PEOPLE LOSE THEIR HAIR?

There are several different reasons why people may begin to lose their hair. It is important to diagnose the cause of your hair loss before you consider which treatment is best for you, as some treatments will only work on certain types of hair loss. Let's have a look at some of the different types of hair loss.

Androgenic Alopecia

Androgenic alopecia, also known as male pattern baldness (MPB), is the most common form of hair loss. Although people refer to it as male pattern baldness, it can occasionally affect women as well.

In general MPB occurs in a similar pattern; hair loss begins by receding at the temples, and hair also thins on the crown. This continues until hair on top of the head disappears completely, leaving hair on just the back and sides of the head. In very rare cases, even these areas can be affected. This type of hair loss is genetic, and can be inherited from either parent.

Now for the scientific part…

MPB is now understood to be related to hormones known as androgens. Androgens are hormones that are important for a number of functions, such as regulating sex drive and regulating hair growth. One of these hormones, dihydrotestosterone (DHT), is primarily responsible for male pattern baldness. This occurs when the hair follicles on people's scalp have a genetic sensitivity to DHT, causing them to shrink. This causes them to have a shorter life span. Understanding this process is the key to understanding how certain treatments work.

Alopecia Areata

This type of hair loss does not generally follow any specific pattern and can occur equally in both men and women. Alopecia areata is relatively common, and hair loss is generally patchy and unpredictable. There is a wide range of possible causes; these can be anything from stress, to an imbalance within a person's body. Luckily, this can generally be determined from a blood test and appropriately treated by a doctor. This type of hair loss will often correct itself in time.

Alopecia Totalis

This is a more severe (and rare) form of alopecia areata, where all or the majority of head hair is lost, including the eyebrows and eyelashes. In extreme cases, all body hair is lost, a condition known as alopecia universalis.

Telogen Effluvium

Telogen Effluvium is characterised by the sudden 'shedding' of hair from the scalp. This is happens when the growth cycle is interrupted by external conditions. This can be down to a large number of reasons, the most common being Chemotherapy and child birth. Other possible causes include illness, infection and severe stress. Whatever the cause is, hair follicles are prematurely pushed from the androgen phase into the telogen phase. As the follicles do not actually die during this type of shedding, telogen effluvium is totally reversible and is generally only temporary.

Now that we understand the different types of hair loss and their causes, let's have a look at some of the common treatments that are available.

4 POPULAR TREATMENTS

In this chapter we'll have a look at some of the common options available for the reversal of hair loss, and how effective they are. So, where better to start than with perhaps the best known solution...

MINOXIDIL

The effects of Minoxidil, often marketed as Rogaine (or Regaine in Europe), on hair loss was an accidental discovery. It was originally used to treat high blood pressure by dilating blood vessels. It was soon discovered that Minoxidil also affected the structure and activity of hair follicles, reactivating previously inactive follicles and therefore stimulating hair re-growth.

How does this work?

The truth is, nobody knows for sure. However, the general accepted theory is that the increase of blood flow around the scalp allows more oxygen to hair follicles, increasing their size to enable them to function again.

How effective is Minoxidil?

Minoxidil can be very effective, certainly one of the most effective options available. However, this does differ from one person to another. Studies have shown that around two thirds of men or women who use Minoxidil will either maintain or increase their hair count. Out of the other third, some will experience slowing in the rate of hair loss, while others will experience no positive effects at all.

Be patient. Often, when people begin using Minoxidil, they are shocked to see their hair loss actually begin to increase over the first few weeks. Don't panic! This is often referred to as the 'dread shed' period and is completely normal. It is in fact a good sign as it shows that the Minoxidil is actually having an effect on the follicles. It happens because follicles that were dying and therefore producing thin hair, are becoming more healthy. They enter the telogen phase, shedding their existing hair in preparation to begin a new growth phase of much thicker hair. Full effects of Minoxidil take between three and twelve months, so patience is required.

Minoxidil can be effective for all types of hair loss.

What are the side effects?

Minoxidil is generally considered to be a very safe product, and serious side effects (dizziness, allergic reactions, difficulty breathing) are very uncommon. If any of these are experienced, it goes without saying that treatment should be stopped immediately. It is extremely unlikely that you will experience anything of this kind.

The most common side effect people experience is itchy scalp. I personally found this to be a problem when I first began using Minoxidil. However, Minoxidil comes in two forms: liquid and foam. Once I switched to the foam, any itching quickly disappeared. Both the liquid and foam contain alcohol, however, which can dry the scalp and cause dandruff. If this does happen, there are anti-dandruff shampoos which can actually help to treat hair loss themselves (as we shall see), so this can be used a good opportunity to combine hair loss treatments in order to maximise effects.

What brands of Minoxidil are available?

For years, Regaine / Rogaine solution was the only brand of Minoxidil available, as the company that makes it (Pfizer) owned the patent. The patent has now expired, and many generic brands have popped up since. As these brands don't have the marketing power of Pfizer, many people are unaware of their existence and therefore still assume Rogaine to be the only brand available, however using lesser known brands can save you massive amounts of money, despite containing exactly the same ingredients!

Unfortunately, only the liquid solution is available in brands other than Rogaine; Pfizer still own the patent on the foam, so for now this form of Minoxidil does work out to be more expensive.

My experience of Minoxidil

I have been using Minoxidil for around nine years now and have always found it to be very effective. As I mentioned before, I prefer to use the foam as I find this results in less irritation to my scalp, but I used the liquid form for several years and found this to be equally as effective. Another benefit I do find from using the foam is that it is easier for apply and spread around the necessary areas; I have moderately lengthy hair, so the liquid is difficult to spread evenly. If you have short hair, or a shaved head, you shouldn't have this problem.

FINASTERIDE

Finasteride was originally developed to treat enlarged prostate in men, under the name Proscar. As it works by reducing the production of DHT, its effects on hair loss quickly became apparent and it became FDA approved as a hair loss treatment in 1997, under the name Propecia.

How does it work?

Finasteride inhibits the production of 'Type II 5-Alpha Reductase' (try saying that when you're drunk!), an enzyme responsible for converting testosterone to DHT. As I mentioned earlier, DHT is the stuff that kills your follicles, so by significantly reducing its presence in your system your follicles are able to continue their happy existence. As a sort of 'thank you', they will reward you with some nice, thick strands of hair to replace the thin or no hair they were producing before.

How effective is Finasteride?

Used only to treat male pattern baldness (in the context of hair loss), Finasteride is extremely effective, having positive effects on nine out of ten men. In studies, over a five year period 48% of men re-grew hair, while 42% experienced no further hair loss during this time.

Finasteride can be used along with Minoxidil for maximum effect. Because they both work in different ways, they complement each other well and allow you to tackle hair loss from two different angles at the same time.

As with Minoxidil, Finasteride takes about three to twelve months to take full effect.

Availability

Finasteride is currently a prescription-only medication (at least in the UK and USA). The patent ran out in 2006, so generic brands are available over the internet. As sites selling these are operating outside of FDA (or MHRA in the UK) guidelines, there is both a legal and possible health risk to buying from them. I therefore do not really want to promote any specific sites or brands that are available for these, however if you're happy to accept these risks, various sellers can easily be found by Googling 'generic Finasteride'

What are the side effects?

Because Finasteride affects androgens, hormones which are related to sexual activity, most possible side effects are sex-related. These can include things such as impotence, decreased libido and abnormal ejaculation. Severe side-effects are relatively uncommon, but if you do experience any of these, by stopping taking the drug you should return to normal.

My experience of Finasteride

I have been taking finasteride for around five years now and have found it to be extremely effective. Although I wasn't visibly balding while I was just using Minoxidil, once I began taking Finasteride I noticed a significant increase in the thickness of my existing hair, and this has remained ever since.

The only side effect I have noticed from taking Finasteride is a decrease in libido. I have had periods of travelling where I have stopped taking Finasteride for a couple of months and it has returned to normal during these times. I don't want to overstate this effect though; without meaning to be too candid, I value my sex life as much as I value my hair, so if the effects had been too severe I wouldn't have continued to take Finasteride for as long as I have.

Warning!

Finasteride has only been demonstrated to be effective on men. Women who are pregnant or anticipate having children any time in the near future should not even handle Finasteride as it can have detrimental effects on pregnancies.

DUTASTERIDE

Dutasteride is currently the most effective hair loss treatment available. It works in much the same was as Finasteride, by inhibiting the Type II 5-Alpha Reductase enzyme, and therefore reducing the amount of follicle-killing DHT. However, the 5-Alpha Reductase enzyme also has a Type I 'version'. While Finasteride has very little effect on this, Dutasteride is very active on both types and therefore reduces DHT even further. Although official case study figures haven't yet been published, Dutasteride has already been demonstrated to be more effective for hair loss than anything else available.

Availability

Unfortunately, at the time of writing this, Dutasteride is not yet approved by either the FDA or the MHRA for the treatment of hair loss. It is, however, approved for the treatment of enlarged prostate (like Finasteride), so it can be prescribed 'off-label' for hair loss at a doctor's disgression. The term 'off-label' is used for when a doctor prescribes a medication in order to treat something other than what the drug is approved for. Therefore, being prescribed Dutasteride is a bit hit and miss.

Studies are currently being done by Glaxosmithkline, the world's second biggest drug company, into Dutasteride's safety with a view to seeking FDA approval as a hair loss treatment in the near future.

What are the side effects?

In unofficial studies, Dutasteride has been shown to have the same side-effects as Finasteride, with pretty much the same likelihood of side-effects occurring.

I personally have had no experience of Dutasteride; as Finasteride has continued to work, I have had no need to. I would recommend attempting to get hold of Dutasteride only if you have tried Finasteride and it hasn't worked. This will more than likely make your doctor more likely to prescribe Dutasteride as a better alternative.

Warning!

As with Finasteride, Dutasteride is for use by men only, and can have the same negative impacts on pregnancies.

KETOCONAZOLE

Ketoconazole is marketed under the brand name Nizoral, and is primarily used as an anti-dandruff shampoo. It is unknown exactly why Ketoconazole works for hair loss. It is speculated, however, that as Ketoconazole kills a type of fungus that naturally inhabits the scalp, this reduces the inflammatory effects of the fungus and therefore promotes hair growth.

How effective is Ketoconazole?

Currently, there have been insufficient studies done on Ketoconazole as a treatment for hair loss in order for the FDA to approve it for this purpose. This doesn't suggest in any way that it doesn't work, only that it hasn't been tested properly – yet. However, it is approved for over-the-counter sales in both the US and UK, so its safety is not in question.

Of the two studies that have been done to demonstrate the efficacy of Ketoconazole as a hair loss treatment, both have found it to have a similar success rate as Minoxidil, making it likely that it is one of the most effective topical treatments available. This was based on men using Nizoral every two to four days.

What are the side effects?

The more common side effects (although not particularly common at all) are nausea or stomach pain / upset. As with any medication, severe side effects are possible but very unlikely. These generally manifest in the form of allergic reactions or burning / itching of the skin. If any of these side effects are experienced, treatment should be stopped.

My personal experience

I have been using Nizoral for around two years now. I have had no adverse effects from it at all. It's difficult to say how well it has been working; my head of hair was already thick when I began using it. However, it does give me the additional peace of mind of tackling hair loss from yet another angle, and at least I don't have to worry about dandruff!

LASERCOMB

The Lasercomb is a device patented and marketed by HairMax. Unsurprisingly, it is a comb with lasers on it. HairMax boast that it is currently the only device that is cleared by the FDA for treatment for hair loss.

How does it work?

The use of lasers has been long since demonstrated to increase the volume of adenosine triphosphate (ATP) in the skin. ATP is a transporter of energy between cells, so more of this stuff can increase cell activity. The hypothetical upshot of this is that this creates more activity in hair follicles, when lasers are used on the scalp.

How effective is the Lasercomb?

This is currently an area of dispute. HairMax have not been particularly forthcoming with the results of their studies, which is never a good sign. Of the study I did manage to find, the differences between the placebo group and the group using the Lasercomb group were minimal and therefore inconclusive.

If results are inconclusive, why have the FDA cleared Lasercomb for hair loss treatment?

This is where the confusion comes in. While HairMax boast about their product's FDA clearance, what they don't do is explain exactly what this means. For a product to be cleared by the FDA, a company must prove its safety for use in the way it's intended to be used. So HairMax obviously demonstrated sufficiently that there have been no adverse effects to people using the Lasercomb for hair loss. This does not, however, mean that the FDA are in any way advocating the use of the Lasercomb as a treatment, only that they have cleared it on the grounds of safety. Once the FDA have seen sufficient evidence to demonstrate a product's effectiveness, they will approve it, and this product is not currently FDA approved, it is only FDA cleared. So while it is obviously a safe product to use, there are no assurances that it actually works. For obvious reasons, HairMax aren't going to want to broadcast this fact too loudly.

I have never used the Lasercomb; it is expensive and therefore not something I considered worthwhile purchasing based on its dubious results. I would personally steer clear of this one for now, unless you have money to burn.

NOURKRIN

Nourkrin is a brand which markets itself as a natural, drug-free treatment for hair loss. Its 'active ingredients' are a mixture of proteins, Vitamin C, Silica and Horsetail Extract.

While all of these ingredients are indeed good for your hair (and skin), there is no actual evidence that any of these products promote hair re-growth. The product boasts exciting statistics regarding studies carried out on the product, although as none of these are confirmed by either the MHRA or FDA, it's really just a case of having to take their word for it.

I have not used Nourkrin personally, however I have spoken with many people who have. While none of these people have reported any hair re-growth from using it, a good proportion of them have reported that their thinning has stopped while they've been using it, and that their existing hair feels healthier.

As no one treatment works for everyone, any hair loss treatment is a punt of sorts. However, Nourkrin comes with a very expensive price tag, with overstated rewards, so it's really up to you to weigh up whether the potential benefits outweigh the damage to your bank account!

5 NATURAL TREATMENTS

While the majority of people seeking hair re-growth opt for one or more of the treatments in the previous chapter, some people prefer to tackle things the natural way. Using chemicals or devices is by no means the only way to promote hair re-growth, and there are plenty of natural options available to do this that many people are unaware of. Some of these can be very effective, and in fact work in similar ways to some of the chemical treatments.

Unfortunately, not as many studies are done on natural treatments as on pharmaceutical options. The reasons for this are obvious: natural treatments are far easier to produce and impossible to patent. For this reason, it is not worth a company's while to spend lots of money investigating the effectiveness of a product that can then be mass-produced by virtually any company that chooses to do it.

It's well worth considering using some natural treatments along with treatments mentioned in the previous chapter; there's a good chance they can enhance the effects, and there's also the added benefit that some of these products are actually good for you in other ways.

There are endless so-called hair loss treatments from natural sources, but the majority have no scientific basis whatsoever, so I've only listed the most credible ones. Let's begin with arguably the most common natural treatment...

SAW PALMETTO EXTRACT

Saw Palmetto extract is an extract of the fruit of Serenoa Repens, a plant that has been used for many years for its medicinal qualities. In the past it has been used as an appetite stimulant and also to treat a variety of conditions such as enlarged prostate, infertility and... yep, you guessed it – hair loss.

Saw Palmetto has been demonstrated to inhibit both types of 5-alpha reductase, therefore working in much the same way as Dutasteride to reduce the amount of DHT in the system, resulting in healthier follicles. Although studies are very limited and usually use very small samples of people, generally they appear to indicate a high success rate with Saw Palmetto when compared to the effects of a placebo.

If you choose to buy Saw Palmetto Extract, to be effective for hair loss the bottle should specify that it is standardised berry extract, with 85% to 95% fatty acids and sterols. General recommended dose is around 320mg daily.

PYGEUM AFRICANUM

Pygeum Africanum is an evergreen tree found in parts of Africa. Extracts of its bark are found to contain high volumes of fatty acids, which have been found (perhaps assumed would be more accurate) to have similar effects on DHT (and therefore hair loss) as Saw Palmetto.

Unfortunately, no studies have been done to prove the efficacy of Pygeum as a hair loss treatment; however there have been many positive testimonies from people using it for this reason over the years. In fact, it is suggested that combining this with Nettle Root Extract (which we'll look at next) for daily use can increase the effectiveness of both herbs.

Recommended dose is 100mg to 200mg daily. Extracts should be standardised to around 13% sterols.

NETTLE ROOT EXTRACT

Once again, Nettle Root Extract is believed to reduce DHT by blocking our beloved 5-alpha reductase enzymes. And, again, as no studies have really been done to test its effects on hair loss, its effectiveness as a treatment is more speculative than anything. However, it has been demonstrated to be effective as a treatment for enlarged prostate, and therefore there is evidence to suggest it would have at least some positive effects as a hair loss remedy.

As I mentioned, advocates of Nettle Root as a hair loss treatment have reported an increased efficacy when combined with Pygeum Africanum extract. Recommended dosage of Nettle Root Extract is typically around 500mg daily.

GREEN TEA

I'm sure you've heard of this one! Aside from being a tasty beverage, there is good evidence to suggest that green tea has a positive effect as a hair loss remedy.

Green tea contains substances known as Polyphenol Catechins. Until recently, it was believe that it was the effect of the polyphenols on DHT that promoted hair re-growth. However, although no studies have been done on people, recently tests were performed on mice. It was found that the anti-inflammatory effects of the polyphenols in green tea were effective in sustaining and re-growing hair in mice, when compared to a control group of mice where no treatment was used.

The problem is, in order to drink enough green tea to be effective as a treatment, you would need to drink about six cups a day, which almost seems like having a full time job. Fortunately, capsules of catechins are available, so this is probably a more practical method of consumption! About 300mg daily is the recommended dose.

Green tea also has a whole range of additional health benefits, so it well worth the 'gamble' as a hair loss treatment.

6 HAIR TRANSPLANTATION SURGERY

Okay, so now we've looked at some of the more preferred treatments available for hair loss, let's have a look at a more drastic form of treatment. Chances are good that one or more of the treatments from the last two chapters will have helped you to regain / keep the full head of hair you've always wanted. However, if all else fails, there is another option.

Hair transplantation works using a process known as FUE – Follicular Unit Extraction. Basically, surgeons extract hair from an area rich in DHT-resistant follicles, generally the back of the head, and implant these into balding areas on the scalp. As we usually have a lot of hair on the backs of our heads, the thinning in the area is unnoticeable, but effects on the appearance of the scalp can be immense.

Obviously the amount of hair that can be transplanted is limited, and therefore it is unlikely that you will end up with a complete head of hair after surgery, however generally patients can expect to see a large portion of their hairline return, to the extent that they will just look to be receding at the temples.

With advances in surgical techniques, recovery time from this type of operation is very quick, with the patient being able to leave the hospital the same day. The surgery generally takes around six to eight hours to complete. Typically between 1500 and 3000 grafts are transplanted.

The effects of the surgery 'shock' the follicles and force them prematurely into the Telogen phase. For this reason, hair re-growth can take up to three months after surgery. So don't go planning any photo shoots for the following weekend! Any scars from the operation should be temporary and will disappear within a week.

The important thing, when considering hair transplantation surgery, is to find the right surgeon. Hair transplantation is nothing less than an art form; the surgeon must transplant in such a way to keep a natural shape of the hairline, as well as transplanting with the direction of hair growth in mind. It is a highly skilled job which, naturally, some people are better at than others.

There are many websites where you can read user reviews comparing individual experiences of treatment. These sites often contains useful forums where people can provide reviews and information about different surgeons around the world, based on their personal experiences.

One thing is for sure – hair transplantation surgery isn't cheap. Prices vary wildly, depending on which surgeon you use, as well as the extent of surgery required. This can be anything from $3 to $10 per graft. If you have a lot of hair loss and would like an experienced surgeon, you would expect to be paying no less than $12,000 for the surgery.

Hair surgery is becoming increasingly popular these days, with celebrities such as Mel Gibson, Jude Law and Kevin Costner all rumoured to have had the operation. So examples of its success rates are all over the net, and well worth checking out if you are considering this option.

7 A HEALTHY LIFESTYLE

Using any of the above treatments will only take you so far towards halting your hair loss. Leading a healthy lifestyle is key to maintaining a good, healthy head of hair.

YOUR DIET

We've all heard the age-old cliché, "You are what you eat". This is as true for hair as it is for any other part of your anatomy. The effect your diet has on the health of your hair should not be underestimated.

Hair is made predominantly of protein, however a good balance of all nutrients is required in order for the various processes involved in producing healthy hair to function well. If your diet is particularly unhealthy, it is much more likely that even the most reliable treatments will fail to help you to retain a healthy head of hair.

A healthy diet should include:

• Fruit & vegetables – Any healthy diet should include five portions of fruit or vegetables a day. These supply your body with fibre and important vitamins and which are important for, among other things, healthy hair. While all vegetables help, ones of the green, leafy variety, such as cabbage and spinach, are particularly recommended for maximum benefit.

• Dairy – Dairy products, such as milk, eggs and cheese, are good sources of the vitamin B-12 as well as protein, both of which promote good hair growth.

• Lean, healthy meats – Things like chicken, fish and organ meats (kidney, liver) are all good sources of vitamins and iron essential to your hair follicles.

• Water – A healthy intake of water is absolutely essential in order to transport important nutrients to hair follicles. You should aim to drink at least 8 glasses of water per day (based on an ounce glass – basically a standard tumbler). Dehydration can have a dramatic effect on the health and volume of your hair, as well as many other things such as skin health and energy levels.

Foods to keep to a minimum:

• Sugar – Too much sugar can speed up the cellular aging process. This can cause a dry scalp, and also hair loss.

• Fatty Foods – Obviously a certain amount of fat is an essential part of any diet. But too much fat can replace the protein that is necessary for hair growth.

• Salt – Too much salt can cause high blood pressure. This can be a problem as a healthy blood supply is essential for maintaining healthy hair follicles.

TOXINS

Toxins, such as alcohol and other drugs, can all have negative effects on hair loss. All toxins have an impact on the body's chemical balance, which can have all sorts of effects, including hair loss. Alcohol, for example, can deplete the body's reserves of zinc; zinc is essential for hair growth, so obviously too much alcohol can have a direct impact on the health of your hair. But don't worry, you don't necessarily need to go teetotal just yet! In moderation alcohol doesn't seem to be a problem, just don't overdo it.

Caffeine, as well, is fine to drink in moderation. However, too much caffeine can cause stress, which in turn can cause hair loss.

Smoking tobacco can damage the DNA of hair follicles, as well as having a negative impact on circulation. Good circulation is very important for a good head of hair, so smoking inevitably is bad for your hair.

Chlorine is a powerful chemical that can adversely affect hair follicles if left on the scalp for too long. If you have been swimming in a chlorinated pool, be sure to have a shower as soon as possible after getting out, in order to rid your skin of the potentially damaging chemical.

Another possible cause of hair loss comes in the form of amalgam fillings. If you have fillings in any of your teeth and they are silver, the chances are they are made from amalgam. Amalgam contains mercury, which is a highly toxic chemical.

There is no actually proof that having amalgam fillings contributes to hair loss, but there is a general feeling among some people that they can have a toxic effect on the body, and in turn, the scalp. Mercury poisoning is known to cause all sorts of health problems, and hair loss is one of them. The debate is whether or not the fillings in your mouth do give off vapours enough to affect you.

Some people have reported hair re-growth after having their amalgam fillings removed. So, if you can, opt for the white fillings next time the dentist tells you you're in need of them. These contain no mercury and will definitely not contribute towards your hair loss.

EXERCISE

A healthy exercise regime can go a long way towards supporting and promoting hair growth. Aerobic exercises, such as jogging, help to wake your body up and increase circulation, which helps to fuel hair follicles with those important nutrients. In short, a certain amount of regular exercise helps to keep you healthy, and the overall health of your body is reflected in the health of your hair.

A huge amount of exercise is not essential; a five to ten minute jog two to three times a week is enough to make a noticeable difference to your health, over time. If you do start exercising heavily, however, you must adjust your diet accordingly – if you do not adjust your diet, heavy exercise can quickly drain your body of important nutrients that are required for hair growth, among other things.

STRESS

Stress is a very common cause of hair loss. None of us can rid ourselves permanently of stress; in fact, stress is an important part of our make up, providing us with, amongst other things, our drive and ambition. But too much stress can be a killer, and one of its victims is the innocent hair follicle.

It's all very well saying "avoid stress where possible", but let's face it, this is an obvious approach even if you're not worried about losing your hair. If you are stressed out, naturally your first step should be to establish to cause of your stress and overcome it, or at least minimise it. But where this isn't possible, there are a couple of other things you can try.

Meditation has been used for centuries to relieve stress. This can be very effective; fitting meditation into your regular routine can work wonders for your health in all sorts of ways, not least of which is stress relief.

Magnesium supplements can also help to relieve stress. When people get stressed, their body's supply of magnesium becomes significantly depleted. Replacing this can go some of the way towards de-stressing (instead of distressing!) you.

8 KEEP YOUR HAIR ON!

If you experiment with the various treatments listed in this book and keep an eye on your lifestyle, there's no reason you can't re-grow and retain a full, healthy head of hair. Here are just a few things to remember in order to help you along your way,,,

Don't Panic!

Even if your treatment is successful, it is likely you will still experience periods where your hair loss seems to have once again reared its ugly head. The key here is not to panic. Apart from the fact that stressing out about it can increase the problem, chances are you actually have nothing to worry about. You may well just have more hair follicles entering their 'resting' phase than normal. If this is the case, your increased hair loss won't last more than a couple of weeks and your hair should have returned to normal within two to three months.

If your hair loss does continue for more than a couple of weeks, consider the following:

• Have you changed your lifestyle? Or do you need a lifestyle change? Read through the previous chapter again and treat it like a checklist. If any area of your lifestyle could be improved, why not try it?

• Have you been dying your hair? With repeated use, hair dyes can sometimes be responsible for triggering hair loss. Using hair straighteners too regularly can have a similar effect. This is completely reversible once you stop using the dye / straighteners.

• If you are happy that your lifestyle isn't the issue, it's possible that your treatment has stopped working. Some people's bodies can build up a natural tolerance to certain treatments, so they become less effective. Don't see this as too much of a problem; as we have seen, there are a good number of options available. If one of them has stopped working, try one or more of the others. Or, if you are using, for example, Minoxidil on its own, try taking Finasteride as well. The combination of Minoxidil and a DHT blocker can give hair loss a double blow.

A Work In Progress

It helps to always think of your hair as a work in progress. Once you start to re-grow the hair you've lost, excitement kicks in and it's easy to think you've cracked it. And to be fair, in a way you have, but don't be too complacent. Stick rigidly to whatever treatment you've been using while it continues to work. But be prepared to alter your ways if you need to.

Medications can work for years and then suddenly stop. Changes in lifestyle can cause you to begin losing hair. Whatever issues occur, be prepared for them and be flexible with how you choose to tackle your hair loss. Be ready to adapt to new circumstances and you will soon feel like you are in control of your hair loss, rather than it being in control of you.

More than anything, be aware of this – whatever treatment you have used to grow back your hair, it will only continue to work for as long as you keep using it. No treatment (with the possible exception of hair transplantation surgery) is designed to tackle the cause of hair loss, only the symptoms. Therefore, if you discontinue treatment, your hair follicles will once again be under attack and within a few short months, you'll be back to square one.

Whatever you do, stay positive. We are now in an age where baldness is no longer an inevitability, and where you can take back control of your hair loss.

Here's to your success!

ALSO AVAILABE BY BEN CRADDOCK:

Self-Publishing Made Easy
A step-by-step guide to conceiving, creating, publishing and
marketing your first e-book